The Root to Rapunzel

Unleashing the Secrets to Luxurious, Lustrous Locks

By

Maria Morgan

Table of Content

Introduction

All of us aspire to have hair as long, strong, and gorgeous as Rapunzel from the Cinderella story. But with so many items, suggestions, and instructions available online, accomplishing that can appear to be an insurmountable challenge. Now that you have "The Root to Rapunzel: Unleashing the Secrets to Luxurious, Lustrous Hair," you can fulfill all of your hair fantasies.

Your go-to resource for developing long, healthy, and natural hair is this book. It is intended to assist you in comprehending the science underlying hair development and to provide you with helpful advice on how to design a personalized hair care routine that is effective for you. This book provides something for everyone, regardless of whether your hair is natural or has had chemical treatment.

The goal of "The Root to Rapunzel" is to grow healthy hair, not only long hair. You'll discover how to feed your body with vital nutrients and a balanced diet to nurture your hair from the inside out.

You will also learn how crucial it is to use natural hair care products and steer clear of chemicals that destroy your hair. The book covers a variety of subjects, including the fundamentals of hair care, hair type and texture, natural hair care, and how to solve typical hair issues. Each topic is thoroughly examined, and the hints and recommendations are supported by professional expertise and scientific study.

In "The Root to Rapunzel," you will uncover the secrets to achieving luscious, lustrous locks. You'll discover how to grow your hair as long as it can and keep it as healthy as you can. The book "The Root to Rapunzel: Unleashing the Secrets to Luxurious, Lustrous Locks" will help you realize the full potential of your hair.

Chapter 1

Learn About The Science Of Hair Growth To Understand How It Develops, What Influences It, And How To Encourage Healthy Development.

A number of stages and other elements go into the biological process of hair growth. To encourage healthy development and reach your hair objectives, it is imperative to understand the science behind hair growth. The many stages of hair growth and the variables that can affect hair growth will be discussed in more detail.

Anagen phase, which is the hair follicle's active growth phase, is the first stage of hair growth. As the hair follicle's cells proliferate and force the hair shaft upward, new hair is created during this period. Genes play a major role in determining the anagen phase's duration, which might vary from person to person. Anagen lasts from two to six years on average.

The catagen phase, which is in between stages, is the second stage of hair development. The hair follicle is getting ready to go into the resting phase at this point. During two to three weeks on average, the catagen phase lasts.

The telogen phase—a resting phase—is the last step of hair development. The hair follicle goes into dormancy at this time, and the hair starts to fall out. The telogen phase lasts, on average, three to four months. The cycle repeats again as the hair follicle enters the anagen phase once more after the telogen period.

Genetics, hormones, nutrition, and stress are just a few of the variables that might affect hair growth. Your hair's length, thickness, and growth rate are all significantly influenced by your genetics. The growth of hair is also influenced by hormones including estrogen and testosterone, with imbalances possibly resulting in hair loss. Nutrition is important for good hair growth because healthy hair is produced by hair follicles, which need crucial nutrients including protein, iron, and biotin. Stress can also affect how quickly hair grows, and long-term stress may even result in hair loss.

There are various things you may do to encourage healthy hair development. It's crucial to get a nutritious diet full of minerals including protein, iron, and biotin. Keeping your hair away from damaging chemical treatments and heat styling can also assist to safeguard it and encourage healthy development. Using hair care items made specifically to nourish and stimulate growth might also be beneficial.

In conclusion, if you want to grow healthy, beautiful hair, you must comprehend the science of hair growth. You may take action to attain your hair objectives and keep your hair healthy for years to come by being aware of the various stages of hair growth, the elements that influence it, and the best ways to encourage healthy growth.

Hair growth-related factors

Hair development is influenced by a wide range of complicated factors. Hormonal changes, food and nutrition, stress and lifestyle, genetics and heredity, diet and nutrition, stress and lifestyle, and environmental variables are some of the most important elements that might affect hair growth.

It's crucial to comprehend these elements if you want to encourage strong hair development and stop hair thinning or loss.

7

Hair growth patterns and traits are greatly influenced by genetics and inheritance. Genetics has a big role in determining characteristics including hair thickness, texture, and color. Understanding your family's history of hair loss might help you take proactive measures to preserve healthy hair, even if there is no way to reverse your genetic tendency to hair thinning or loss. The development of hair can also be greatly impacted by hormonal changes. Estrogen and testosterone are two examples of hormones that can alter hair development cycles and result in hair loss or thinning. The considerable hormonal changes that occur throughout puberty, pregnancy, and menopause can all have an impact on hair growth. It's crucial to comprehend these changes and how they affect hair development if you want to keep your hair healthy.

Nutrition and diet are also very important for hair development. A nutritious diet high in vitamins, minerals, and protein helps support the growth of good hair. For healthy hair, nutrients like biotin, vitamin D, and iron are particularly crucial.

Healthy hair development can be aided by eating a balanced diet, vitamins, and a healthy lifestyle. Lifestyle decisions and stress may both affect hair growth. Stress and lifestyle choices like smoking and drinking alcohol can also result in hair loss or thinning. Positive stress management practices and abstaining from bad behaviors can support healthy hair development.

Hair growth may also be impacted by environmental variables such air pollution, climate, and water quality. Damage from the environment can make hair dry, brittle, and prone to breaking. When required, covering hair and using preventive measures to protect it from environmental harm can aid in promoting healthy hair development.

The use of certain drugs and medical conditions might also have an impact on hair growth. Hair loss or thinning can be brought on by a number of medical illnesses, including thyroid disorders, autoimmune diseases, and ailments of the scalp like psoriasis. Hair loss can also be brought on by several treatments, particularly chemotherapy drugs. The possible negative effects of any drugs you are taking should be understood, and you should consult your doctor if you notice hair thinning or loss.

Hair care habits might affect hair development as well. Hair damage causes it to break or fall out and can be brought on by over-washing, excessive heat style, and harsh chemical treatments. Utilizing mild hair care products, staying away from harsh chemicals and heat styling tools, and protecting hair during styling can all aid in promoting healthy hair development.Another element that may affect hair growth is age. Hair follicles may become less active as we age, which may cause hair loss or thinning. As we age, maintaining overall health and wellbeing via regular exercise, a balanced diet, and stress management can help preserve good hair.

In conclusion, a variety of factors, including genetics, hormones, food, nutrition, stress, lifestyle, environmental factors, medical problems, medicines, hair care routines, and age, can impact hair development. It is possible to encourage healthy hair development and keep strong, luscious locks by being aware of these variables and taking action to solve any problems.

Chapter 2

What Is Your Hair Type: What Texture and Kind of Hair Do You Have?

Each person has a different hair type and texture. To find the hair care methods that are right for you, it is crucial to understand your hair type and texture. This chapter will discuss several hair kinds and how to determine your own hair type and texture.

Hair can be classified as straight, wavy, or curly. Compared to wavy or curly hair, straight hair is normally smooth and lustrous and tends to be oilier. When compared to straight hair, wavy hair has a modest wave or curl pattern and greater body and substance. A variety of curl patterns, from loose curls to tight coils, are characteristic of curly hair. The thickness or diameter of each individual hair strand is referred to as hair texture. Typically, hair textures are categorized as fine, medium, or coarse. Coarse hair strands are robust and solid, whereas fine hair strands are fragile and thin. Hair that is in the middle falls somewhere in between.

Observing your hair's natural texture, curl pattern, and thickness will help you determine your hair type and texture. By taking a strand of your hair and attentively analyzing it, you may establish the type and texture of your hair. You have straight hair if it is reasonably straight and rests flat against your head. You have wavy hair if it has a gentle wave or curl pattern. You have curly hair if it has a noticeable curl pattern. Run a strand of hair between your fingers to assess the texture of your hair. You have fine hair if you can hardly feel a hair strand. You have medium hair if you can feel the hair strand. You have coarse hair if a hair strand feels thick and coarse. You may modify your hair care regimen to meet your demands once you've determined your hair type and texture. Those with thin hair, for instance, should stay away from heavy hair products that could weigh them down, while people with curly hair should use treatments that highlight and emphasize their natural curl pattern.

The first step to getting healthy, luscious locks is to understand your hair type and texture. Hair can further be categorized as oily, dry, or normal in addition to the three major classifications and three textures. Sebum tends to be overproduced by oily hair, which can leave the hair looking greasy and flat. Natural oils are absent from dry hair, which may cause it to seem drab, brittle, and prone to breakage. Normal hair seems healthy and lustrous and has a balanced oil production.

Genetics, age, hormonal changes, and external elements including environmental toxins, heat styling, and chemical treatments are other variables that can impact hair type and texture. For instance, hormonal changes can affect the texture and thickness of hair, while aging might make it thinner, drier, and more brittle. It is crucial to select hair care items that are especially suited to your hair type once you have identified your hair type and texture. For instance, if you have oily hair, you should seek light, oil-free products that will help you reduce the amount of oil your hair produces. Use moisturizing goods to moisturize and nourish your hair if you have dry hair.

You may pick the best hair care regimen and products to help you obtain healthy, luscious locks by being aware of your hair type and texture. The information and resources in this chapter will provide you the knowledge and skills you need to determine the type and texture of your hair and create a hair care regimen that is right for you.

Chapter 3

Washing, Conditioning, and Styling: The Basics of a Hair Care Regimen

To encourage hair development and avoid damage, it's critical to keep the scalp clean and in good condition. This is why it's so crucial to routinely wash and condition your hair. While conditioning helps to nourish and protect your hair, washing your hair helps to get rid of product buildup, excess oil, and grime.

The proper products for your hair type should be used when washing and conditioning your hair. For instance, a clarifying shampoo might assist to get rid of buildup and extra oil if you have oily hair. In order to hydrate your hair if you have dry hair, you might want to use a moisturizing shampoo and conditioner.

Using the proper method when washing and conditioning your hair is also crucial. This entails distributing the materials evenly and gently massaging your scalp to increase blood flow and encourage strong hair growth.

Also, it's crucial to carefully rinse the product out of your hair to guarantee that none remains. It's crucial to use gentle techniques while styling your hair to prevent damage. To prevent heat damage, this entails avoiding tight hairstyles that might tug on your hair and using heat styling equipment sparingly. Using the proper hair care products, such as leave-in conditioners and heat protectant sprays, is also crucial to preventing damage to your hair. To maintain healthy hair, there are a few more considerations in addition to utilizing the proper tools and methods for washing, conditioning, and style. For instance, it's crucial to refrain from over-washing your hair because doing so might rob your scalp of its natural oils, resulting in dryness and damage. Depending on your hair type and lifestyle, experts advise washing your hair every two to three days.

The temperature of the water you use to wash your hair is another crucial aspect to take into account. While bathing in hot water may seem soothing, doing so might harm your hair by depriving it of its natural oils and resulting in dryness. To help seal your hair cuticles and enhance shine, experts advise washing your hair in lukewarm or cool water and rinsing with cool water afterward.

Because they are the oldest and most vulnerable component of your hair, the ends need special care during conditioning. Adding conditioner to your hair's ends might aid in avoiding split ends and damage. Moreover, once a week deep conditioning treatments might assist to hydrate and strengthen your hair.

Lastly, it's essential to shield your hair from environmental stresses like pollution and sun exposure. Wearing a helmet or scarf helps protect your hair from the sun, and using an oil or serum can screen it from pollution and other environmental elements. You can keep your hair healthy, strong, and shiny for years by following these hair-care instructions. In general, keeping healthy and glossy locks requires adequate hair washing, conditioning, and style. You may obtain the hair of your dreams by using the appropriate products and styling methods, being careful with your hair, and encouraging healthy development.

Chapter 4

The Function of Lifestyle and Diet in Fostering Healthy Hair Development

The food you consume has a big impact on how healthy your hair grows. A protein called keratin, which is created in the hair follicles, makes up your hair. It's crucial to have a balanced diet that gives your body the nutrients it needs to generate keratin and promote healthy hair development if you want your hair to grow and stay healthy.

Protein, iron, zinc, biotin, and vitamins A, C, and E are some of the most important nutrients for promoting healthy hair development. Many foods, such as lean meats, fish, eggs, nuts, seeds, whole grains, and leafy green vegetables, provide these nutrients. A balanced diet and the use of certain supplements can both aid in the promotion of healthy hair development. For instance, studies on certain people have indicated that biotin supplementation can increase hair growth and decrease hair loss. Iron, zinc, vitamins D and B12, and other dietary supplements may also assist healthy hair development.

A lot of lifestyle choices can support healthy hair development in addition to eating a balanced diet and taking supplements. For instance, frequent exercise can enhance scalp circulation and encourage the development of healthy hair. Deep breathing exercises, yoga, and other stress-reduction techniques can lessen hair loss and encourage healthy hair growth. You may encourage healthy hair development and enjoy strong, glossy locks for years to come by paying attention to your diet, taking vitamins as needed, and establishing good lifestyle practices.

While diet and supplements can assist healthy hair development, it's vital to remember that they do not provide a panacea for hair loss or other problems relating to the hair. Genetics, hormonal imbalances, drug side effects, and certain medical problems are just a few of the causes of hair loss. A healthcare professional or hair expert should be consulted if you are having hair loss or other hair-related problems in order to identify the underlying reason and create an effective treatment strategy.

It's crucial to concentrate on nutrient-dense meals that are abundant in the critical vitamins and minerals stated above when trying to incorporate healthy foods into your diet to promote hair development. Many illustrations of good diets for hair development include:

- Lean meats that are rich in protein, iron, and zinc include chicken, turkey, and beef.
- Fatty fish that are strong in omega-3 fatty acids, like salmon and sardines, encourage the formation of good hair.
- Nuts and seeds, particularly those high in biotin and vitamin E like almonds, walnuts, and pumpkin seeds
- leafy green veggies with a high iron, vitamin A, and vitamin C content, like spinach and kale
- Healthy grains that are rich in B vitamins and promote healthy hair development include brown rice and quinoa.

In addition to eating well and taking supplements, there are certain hair care procedures that can encourage the growth of healthy hair. For instance, avoiding overheating styling tools and chemical treatments, routinely washing your hair with a mild shampoo, and using a deep conditioning treatment once per week can all assist to maintain strong, healthy hair.

Chapter 5

The Top Ingredients for Healthy Hair: What to Use and What to Avoid in Natural Goods

As individuals become more aware of the substances they use to their hair and scalp, natural hair care products are growing in popularity. Natural elements used for generations to nourish hair and encourage healthy hair development, such as plant extracts, essential oils, and herbs, are employed in these products.

The fact that natural hair care products don't include damaging chemicals like sulfates, parabens, and synthetic perfumes that can injure hair and irritate the scalp is one of its main advantages. Aloe vera, coconut oil, argan oil, and shea butter are examples of natural nutrients that moisturize and hydrate hair while also encouraging hair development and fortifying hair follicles.

Your hair and general health can both benefit from using natural hair care products. Natural hair care products are manufactured with natural components that are kinder to your hair and scalp than typical hair care products, which might include harsh chemicals and synthetic smells.

Using natural hair care products has certain advantages, such as:

- Better Hair: Natural ingredients like aloe vera, shea butter, and coconut oil may moisturize and nourish your hair, reducing breakage and split ends.
- Less Allergy Reaction: As natural hair care solutions are frequently devoid of harsh chemicals, those with sensitive skin or allergies should choose for them.
- Environmentally Friendly: Biodegradable materials and packaging are frequently used to make natural hair care products, making them a more environmentally friendly option.

The following are some of the top organic components for healthy hair:

- Coconut oil: This organic oil has the ability to penetrate the hair shaft, strengthening and hydrating the hair while preventing protein loss. Coconut oil, which is high in fatty acids, may penetrate the hair shaft to deeply condition and nourish it.

- Shea butter: A natural moisturizer that helps calm dry or irritated scalps and help prevent breakage and split ends. Shea butter, a natural conditioner that is rich in vitamins A and E, can help heal damaged hair and stop breakage.

- Aloe vera: This organic plant extract, which is full of vitamins and minerals, can assist to encourage the growth of healthy hair and calm sensitive scalps. Aloe vera, which is well-known for its hydrating and calming qualities, is a common component in many natural hair care products.

- Argan oil: An all-natural oil rich in important fatty acids and antioxidants, argan oil helps moisturize and nourish hair while shielding it from harm. Vitamin E and antioxidants found in abundance in this oil can help protect hair from harm and encourage the growth of healthy hair.

Avoiding substances that may affect your hair or general health is vital while shopping for natural hair care products. Ingredients to stay away from include:

- Sulfates: These harsh detergents can dry out and irritate your hair by robbing it of its natural oils.
- These preservatives, known as parabens, have been connected to a number of malignancies and can interfere with hormonal balance.
- Synthetic fragrances: They have been related to reproductive problems and can irritate the skin and create allergic responses.

You may support the growth of healthy, gorgeous hair by selecting natural hair care products that are devoid of damaging substances and high in nourishing, natural components. As individuals become more aware of the substances they use to their hair and scalp, natural hair care products are growing in popularity. Natural elements used for generations to nourish hair and encourage healthy hair development, such as plant extracts, essential oils, and herbs, are employed in these products.

The fact that natural hair care products don't include damaging chemicals like sulfates, parabens, and synthetic perfumes that can injure hair and irritate the scalp is one of its main advantages. Aloe vera, coconut oil, argan oil, and shea butter are examples of natural nutrients that moisturize and hydrate hair while also encouraging hair development and fortifying hair follicles.

Chapter 6

Holistic Hair Care: Looking After Your Hair From the Inside Out

Our hair's health can be significantly impacted by our mental wellbeing. Hair loss and thinning can be caused by stress, worry, and despair. On the other hand, taking care of oneself might benefit the condition of one's hair. This chapter examines the relationship between mental health and good hair and offers advice on how to take care of oneself for healthy hair.

Taking care of your hair from the inside out is part of a comprehensive approach to hair care. This includes feeding your body nutritious food, obtaining enough rest, and controlling stress. Iron, biotin, and vitamin D are just a few of the vitamins and minerals that can help support healthy hair development. The importance of getting adequate sleep cannot be overstated. Maintaining stress-free hair requires good stress management. Inflammation brought on by stress might result in hair loss. Exercise, yoga, and other stress-relieving practices can help you control your stress levels.

In addition to caring for your health, it's crucial to take good care of your hair by avoiding harsh chemicals and using natural treatments. Natural components can help feed your hair and encourage healthy development, such as coconut oil, aloe vera, and avocado. Avoid over-styling your hair with hot tools or tight hairstyles, which can lead to breakage and damage.

Improved hair growth and texture, greater self-assurance, and enhanced general health and well-being are just a few advantages of a holistic approach to hair care.

Natural Hair Masks & Treatments for Healthy Hair: At-Home Hair Care

DIY hair treatments have become more and more popular over time as consumers seek for cheap, natural alternatives to costly salon services. These remedies are an excellent choice for folks on a budget because they are not only simple to produce but also contain natural components that are easily found at home. In this article, we'll talk about the advantages of DIY hair treatments and offer some easy-to-use home remedies for hair masks and treatments.

Pros of Do-It-Yourself Hair Treatments

- Affordable: Homemade hair treatments may be produced for a reasonable price using products that are already in the house. They are therefore a great choice for anyone who wishes to reduce their spending on hair care products.

- Natural Ingredients: Chemical-free natural components are used in homemade hair treatments. This indicates that they have no negative effects and are kind to the hair and scalp.
- DIY hair treatments may be made to suit your individual hair demands since they are adaptable. To treat any particular issues like dryness, frizz, or dandruff, you can utilize products that are ideal for your hair type.
- Simple to prepare: The majority of DIY hair treatments are simple to prepare and only need a few components. These treatments are simple to produce at home and don't require any special hair knowledge.

Hair Masks & Treatments to Try at Home That Are Easy and Effective

- Hair mask using coconut oil: A fantastic natural substance that can help hydrate and nourish the hair is coconut oil. Warm up a spoonful of coconut oil and massage it into your scalp and hair to create a coconut oil hair mask. For optimal effects, cover your hair with a shower cap and use it for an hour or overnight.

- Honey and banana hair mask: Hair may be strengthened and nourished by the vitamins and minerals found in bananas, which are abundant in. Natural humectants like honey can help the hair maintain moisture. Blend one ripe banana with two teaspoons of honey to make this mask, then use it on your hair. Before washing it off with water, let it sit for 30 minutes.
- Rinsing with apple cider vinegar can help balance the pH of the scalp and get rid of buildup in the hair. Use this rinse as your last rinse after washing your hair by combining one tablespoon of apple cider vinegar with one cup of water.

How to Establish a Routine for Natural Hair Care

- Choose natural hair care products: Go for hair care items devoid of damaging chemicals like silicones, sulfates, and parabens. Seek for all-natural components that can help nourish and preserve the hair, such as shea butter, argan oil, and coconut oil.

- Less frequent hair washing helps prevent the loss of natural oils that prevent dryness and breakage. To maintain your hair clean and healthy, try to wash it every two to three days.
- Use a wide-toothed comb: A wide-toothed comb can assist in detangling hair without breaking it. Beginning at the ends, begin combing your way up to the roots.
- Avoid using heat styling equipment on your hair since they might promote dryness and brittleness. All heat styling equipment should be used with a heat protectant spray beforehand, and excessive use should be avoided.

Hence, Homemade hair treatments are a fantastic approach to take care of your hair organically and economically. They may be tailored to match your unique hair demands and contain natural ingredients that are kind to the hair and scalp. Including a natural hair care routine in your routine will help you maintain attractive, strong, and healthy hair.

Conclusion

It's crucial to consider the most important lessons you learnt after reading a book on hair care to make sure you're incorporating them into your regular hair care practice. This article will summarize the key ideas from the book, offer encouragement to keep going on your hair care journey, and offer some last thoughts on having healthy, attractive hair.

- Knowing your hair type is important for choosing the best hair care regimen. It's important to know your hair type and use products that are appropriate for it since various hair types demand different care and treatment.
- Healthy Diet: A vitamin and nutrient-rich diet helps encourage healthy hair development. A balanced diet that includes things like salmon, eggs, and leafy greens will help you keep your hair healthy.
- In order to keep healthy hair, a regular hair care routine is necessary. This entails routinely washing your hair, using the appropriate hair care products, and avoiding excessive heat styling.
- In order to keep your hair healthy, it's important to protect it from environmental toxins, heat styling, and chemical treatments. Hair damage may be minimized by using protective hair treatments, avoiding harsh chemicals, and using low heat style.

Inspiration to Keep On on Your Hair Care Journey

Patience, reliability, and commitment are necessary for maintaining good hair. Despite obstacles and disappointments, it's critical to keep going with your hair care regimen. Always keep in mind that having beautiful, healthy hair is possible with the appropriate routine and care.

Lasting Ideas for Growing Healthy, Gorgeous Hair

A holistic strategy that incorporates good nutrition, a healthy hair care regimen, and damage prevention is needed to achieve healthy, gorgeous hair. Everyone can have gorgeous, healthy hair with the proper care and commitment. You'll immediately see the effects of your efforts if you're careful, persistent, and patient with your hair.